Bipolar Disorder in This Up and Down World

Bonnie L. Bair

Galesburg, Illinois

Names: Bair, Bonnie L. | Bair, Bonnie L. editor

Title: Bipolar Disorder in This Up and Down World

Description: 1st Edition | Galesburg, Illinois: Life Improvements 2, 2021

Identifiers: LCCN 2021904824

ISBN: 978-0-9994772-3-6

This book is dedicated to all people with a
mental health diagnosis.

Bipolar Disorder in This Up and Down World

Foreword

Society has been so ignorant about bipolar disorder - what to do about it and the judgment of someone with bipolar disorder. It has been grave. Overcoming the stigma can seem insurmountable.

As a retired counselor of over 20 years and an individual diagnosed with bipolar disorder, I felt it important to write about bipolar disorder; to help educate and lessen the stigma society has had about bipolar disorder and offer suggestions for recognizing and adequately dealing with bipolar disorder.

According to the National Institute of Mental Health, over 5 million American adults have bipolar disorder. I venture to guess this number is an underrepresentation of the real number of individuals who have the disease, due to many people going undiagnosed and self-medication.

Chapter 1

What is Bipolar Disorder?

Bipolar disorder is characterized by extremes in highs and lows for an individual in which the person easily cries, laughs, or becomes angry.

Individuals with bipolar disorder have a greater sensitivity to stimuli and stressors such as their own emotions, emotions/behavior of others, environment, world events, etc.

Because individuals with bipolar disorder tend to be acutely in tune with their feelings, they are also acutely in tune and affected by the emotions and judgments of others. This makes them overwhelmed because they are sensitive to environmental and emotional stressors/information. They can feel the pain of others – not just comprehend or understand the pain of others. Many people turn to alcohol or drug use, to deal with the stress and anxiety this causes.

Individuals who have personally struggled with bipolar disorder tend to be intelligent, creative, and compassionate. They are prone to worry, have ADHD or ADD type symptoms, have racing thoughts, may have difficulty with memory, anxiety, time management, or time awareness. They tend to be sensitive to tags in the back of their shirts and sensitivities to uncomfortable clothing such as belts or socks, etc., and can have sudden changes in mood/behavior/sleep patterns/energy level.

Time changes in the spring and fall can create difficulties for individuals with bipolar disorder.

They may tend to want to escape or getaway, by driving or spending money at times of high stress. Some may tend toward work-a-holism, alcoholism, over-eating, drug usage, etc. Each person is different. It depends on their morals. Some may have an overactive sex drive and become involved in pornography. Others may become very spiritual and work harder and harder to do the right things. It depends on the person and their values. During times of stress, others can see behavior changes in them. The changes may include a higher level of confidence or anger, due to injustice or repeated injustices or from others being judgmental. There is also a tendency, as with anyone else, of not having as good of decision-making ability when under times of extreme stress.

Early indicators of the disease: intolerance in wearing tight clothing or clothing with tags.

Individuals may unknowingly self-medicate with drugs or alcohol to stabilize their moods, especially those who regularly use alcohol - as the use of alcohol is accepted and often encouraged in society.

Individuals with bipolar disorder may feel judged by others and feel more inadequate, overwhelmed, frustrated, and angry when others don't understand them.

If someone is in a relationship that feels like a rollercoaster ride, one or both involved may have bipolar disorder. Individuals with bipolar disorder can become bored easily. Therefore, at times they may unconsciously create drama out of boredom.

Individuals with bipolar disorder may have alcohol or drug addictions, spending or gambling problems, inappropriate or many relationships, high Irritability, or work-a-holism. It depends on the person, their personality, and upbringing.

There are 2 different types of bipolar disorder.

1. During a manic episode, the individual may experience delusional thinking /or paranoia. (Usually bipolar 1 disorder)

2. During a depressive episode, the individual may experience suicidal thinking or make suicide attempts. (Usually bipolar 2 disorder)

Chapter 2

If Bipolar Disorder is Suspected

It is important to see a psychiatrist for accurate diagnosis and treatment, especially if another family member has it. Improper or inadequate treatment of bipolar disorder can be dangerous. Regular medical doctors do not have as much schooling as psychiatrists and do not always accurately identify or treat bipolar disorder. There are different treatment options depending on whether a person has bipolar **1** disorder or bipolar **2** disorder. For instance, treating someone who has bipolar **1** disorder with a regular anti-depressant, can make things worse. A mood-stabilizing medication or substance is necessary, instead.

In addition, it's important to communicate clearly and follow up with medical professionals; especially when a person is not feeling well. Each person is different and may respond differently to medications.

Bipolar disorder always requires some medication or nutrients to support the body. Treatment will depend on the individual and on the type of bipolar disorder they have. Bipolar disorder tends to become problematic when a person is in their early to middle '20s. It tends to get worse with age and at times of stress. It needs regular treatment, in some way, for the person to function at their best and for living and have happy relationships.

Chapter 3

Managing Bipolar Disorder

It is very important for individuals with bipolar disorder to get adequate regular sleep (7-12 hours per night). Getting less than needed, can put the person into a "tail-spin" and cause a manic episode. Eating healthy regular meals is also important. Skipping meals can also trigger mania in some individuals. Getting moderate exercise, having daily quiet time, and having a routine with variety (to prevent boredom) is also helpful. Keeping the number of activities and expectations to a minimum, especially during times of stress, is essential. Keeping a list of things to do, at times of boredom, is also helpful.

Medications

Various medications treat bipolar disorder. Although an individual may feel like they don't need medication every day, it's important to support the body with medication and or nutrients daily. It's important for dealing with unexpected stressors. It's like having a surge protector for your computer during a storm. The medicine and/or nutrients act as a surge protector and help with stability when the unexpected stressors of life come. With them continually in the body, the individual will cope and function better. With them, they are more likely to avoid hospitalizations. Seek assistance from a Psychiatrist for medication management.

Nutrients that can help with symptoms of bipolar disorder

Magnesium – It has been depleted in the food supply, due to the use of pesticides and chemicals. Most individuals do not get an adequate supply of magnesium in their diet. Magnesium can help to reduce anxiety and depression.

Vitamin D – Vitamin D is often low in individuals who do not get adequate sun exposure - especially during the winter months. Adequate intake of Vitamin D can help to reduce depression.

Omega 3's – Flax or Fish Oil can help with neurotransmitters for adequate brain function.

Ashwagandha – It's an adaptogen herb that can help a person deal with stress. It can also help with depression, stabilize mood, and help with memory and the ability to handle distractions. It should not be taken by anyone who is allergic to sweet potatoes nor should it be taken by pregnant women.

CBD – It's the form of marijuana that does NOT contain THC (the hallucinogenic property). CBD can help manage anger and stabilize mood. It is not recommended for pregnant women.

Lithium Orotate – It's available over the counter at nutrition stores in 5 or 10 mg amounts. It helps to stabilize mood. It should not be taken with aspirin, naproxen, or Advil, because it can hurt the kidneys.

L-methyl folate – It's been found that some people cannot adequately utilize folic acid and are more susceptible to mental illness. L-methyl folate is an elemental easily absorbed form of folic acid.

Melatonin – Melatonin can help regulate sleep cycles. It is intended for short-term use.

*Nutrients should be thoroughly researched and discussed with medical professionals before taking them. Dosages per individual and interactions with medications will vary. It is helpful to cross-reference the nutrient with the health conditions of concern (or medicine) when researching.

Chapter 4

Dealing with Bipolar Episodes

It is best to prepare for dealing with manic/depressive episodes. Family and friends of individuals with bipolar disorder might feel inadequate and scared because they don't know how to help or what to do. Remember, you can simply let the other person know you care and ask them how you can help. Being willing to do something for them in exchange for them getting help and taking their medication and or nutrients can be helpful. It may be helpful for someone to accompany them to doctor appointments, for complete information sharing with health providers for adequate medicine management. Education, and an atmosphere of understanding, love, and acceptance, will help the most.

Dealing with Manic/Depressive Episodes Reference Sheet

Manic/Depressive episodes can be very stressful for, not only the person experiencing them but also the family and friends of the individual. Instructions for family/friends to follow during these stressful times can help manage the severity and duration of the episodes.

Each person should have a reference sheet for their family and close friends to follow in the case of an emergency.

Here is an example reference sheet is done by someone who has bipolar disorder to help their family deal with them during a manic or depressive bipolar episode:

Sample Notes to Follow for Family/Friends of Individual with Bipolar Disorder

> If you think you ever may be worried about where I am or my safety, ask to add me to your google locator so you know where I am at any time.

Here are the ways you can be helpful to me:

1) Remember: Listen to understand - Not to Judge. Look for and acknowledge the good.
2) Also, remember to be kind and truthful.

OPTIONS:

-Ask if there is something I need.

-Ask if there is something you can pray with me about.

-Ask if you can help by running an errand or helping get medicine/nutrients, or food.

-Ask if I've been sleeping ok, or if I have had their thyroid checked lately.

-Ask if something has happened that I'd like to talk about.

-If you don't understand why I said or did something, ask! Don't jump to conclusions and label me as crazy, just because you don't understand.

-If you feel I'm so stressed that I need something extra to help me, ask me to take a lithium orotate.

- Ask if I'm feeling particularly overwhelmed or angry at someone for something unfair or wrong that they did to me or to someone I care about.

- Ask if there is anything you can do to help me.

- Hug me and tell me you love me.

During the spring and fall (around the time change) Include me by asking me to do something fun with you. Don't add unnecessary responsibilities to me at these times.

*Gentle is best with me. I don't need policemen. I don't need criticism. I don't need to be treated like a sub-par human being, because I may have a health condition that you may be biased against, afraid of, or don't understand.

I need understanding and cooperation.

- If you want me to remember or consider something, just ask. "Would you be willing to...?" will probably work just fine.

- If I'm talking about my feelings more than you are comfortable with, tell me you are feeling overwhelmed. I will gladly find someone else to talk with. I don't want to burden anyone.

I want to be approachable and be able to discuss things with you. I would expect the same respect you or anyone else would. The techniques above will help things to go more smoothly. Please do your best, to be honest, while loving with me. Talking behind my back, excluding me, or making decisions for me or decisions that directly affect me without talking with me will make things much worse for me. Another way I ask that you respect me as a person is that you <u>do not</u> patronize or lie to me. I will be aware of it, and this also will make things much worse for both of us.

Thank you for your love and concern for me. I want to be a blessing and not a curse to you. The things on this sheet will help me to have less anger, be healthier, and be more of a blessing to myself and others. Thank you for taking the time to read it and understand.

Check for further helps in my "Wellness Box." It is located on the dresser next to my bed.

Chapter 5

The Wellness Box

A wellness box is helpful in adequately managing bipolar disorder. It should contain the following:

1. Regular and preventative medications

2. Nutrients

3. Doctor's names and phone numbers

4. Names of friends and phone numbers

5. Notes for staying on track, like:

    a. Affirmations,

    b. Dealing with anger reference notes

    c. Communication helps

6. Reference sheet for family/friends

7. Emergency Plan in case of crisis

Family/Friends should know where the "Wellness Box" is located, so they can have access to it if needed. (Copies of the reference sheet and emergent plan should be given to family/friends ahead of time.)

Having a wellness box to remind the individual with bipolar disorder of important things, is helpful during stressful times and is optimal for maintaining personal health and sanity in relationships. Some of the things it can include: nutrients, medicine, and melatonin (for sleep), phone numbers and resources for friendship and help in times of need, scriptures, affirmations, 2 and 4 step communication techniques, reminders regarding sleep, exercise, variety with routine, food, extra vitamin D between fall and springtime changes, Medical reminders on doctor appointments, thyroid, magnesium, copper level checks, etc. It can also contain reminders about lessening activities and responsibilities around spring and fall time changes and regarding balance in schedule and activities for balance in life and relationships.

It can be kept anywhere that is easy to see and reference, such as on a dresser by the bedside.

It should contain an easy 3-5 step plan to follow in the case of a manic or depressive episode.

For example:

*In the case of mania or depression: 1. Pray with me. 2. Ask me to specifically increase a certain type of medication or nutrient and go to sleep. 3. Schedule an appointment with my doctor. 4. Encourage me to talk with a close friend or counselor about stressors.

It can also contain communication strategy notes for own and family reference: Using these techniques may help with more difficult conversations.

For example:

Two-Step Communication Techniques

"I feel …. (word-not a thought).
"I like when…. or don't like when……"
OR
"I need ………, or would like…"
"Would you be willing to …….?"
OR

I'm thinking you are thinking ……. Is that what you are thinking?

I'm thinking you are feeling …… Is that what you are feeling?

*Four-Step Communication Technique:

1. "I feel ……. (Feeling word)

2. "I like or don't like when ……."

3. "I need or would like ………."

4. "Would you be willing to…….?"

Try to avoid words like: "should, always, never, everything," & "BUT."

Instead, use words like: "sometimes, seldom, often" and "AND."

Additional Notes to keep in Wellness Box for Individual Reference

Ways to Stop Excessive Working, Spending, Eating, TV, Hoarding, Gaming, Addictions, Etc.

by Bonnie Bair of Life Improvements, PLLC, 2019

Seek information about the issue: Talk to God & Ask for Wisdom from God who gives liberally to those who ask. Google the issue. Talk/Listen to someone who cares. Doctor or Expert. Read a Book.

Ask yourself: How much of this excess is due to worry?

1. Pray whenever worried about something & ask God for help
2. Gentle Kegels, with any worry thoughts
3. Omega 3's like hemp, flax, or fish oil; along with Ashwagandha or Holy Basil.
4. Affirmations

Ask Yourself: How much of this is due to loneliness?

1. Pray
2. Consider: getting a roommate or pet, calling someone to see how they are and asking if you can help them with something, or asking a friend (or someone you like) to do something with you, can help

Ask Yourself: How much of this is due to stress?

1. Pray

2. Assess the Source of Stress.

> If Clutter: De-clutter! Look for the easiest thing to start with, then the next, and keep going. Take breaks as you need.

> If too many things to do: Prioritize. Start with the most logical or easiest. Delegate. Ask for help. Change plans or target date.

> If too much information: Read or deal with one thing at a time. Consider fasting Facebook, the news, TV, or

radio. Unsubscribe to unnecessary email. Consider reading, or asking for, a summary of the information sought.

If someone is causing you stress: Talk with them. Ask for cooperation. If they are unwilling, spend less time with them. Spend more time with friends/family who comforts and encourage you. Practice gentle Kegels or belly breathing w stress.

Ask Yourself: How much is due to problems in my relationships?

1. Pray. Ask God for what you want and need.
2. Do Research: Bible, Google, "We Smile" book.
3. Repent/Repair.

Ask Yourself: How much of this is due to boredom?

1. Pray and ask God for an idea or direction.
2. Consider: Creating a list of things to do for reference at times when you get bored. calling a friend or family member and seeing how they are,

taking up a hobby, clearing out the cupboards, doing something for someone else, reading something, or researching something.

Ask Yourself: How much of this is due to <u>sadness</u>?

1. Talk to God.
2. Consider: Telling yourself the truth. Kegels. Align your speech with scripture. Feel the sadness, so it will dissipate. Take a bath. Massage your feet. Talk with a friend or a Counselor. Do some activity that will increase endorphins. Listen to some uplifting or energetic music. Say affirmations. Encourage/Listen to someone else. Watch a movie or something funny. Get some rest. Do something different or interesting. Join a support group.
3. Research nutrients to support your body – Omega 3's, Ashwagandha, Vitamin D, Magnesium, CBD, and L-methyl folate.
4. Talk to your Doctor. Consider medicine. Do your research. Report any concerns to the doctor right away for medicine change

or adjustment. Follow-up with Doctor/Counselor.

Ask Yourself: How much of this is due to my physical health?

1. Pray and ask for wisdom. Ask elders of the church to anoint w/oil and pray for you.
2. Do research. Google how to treat the condition
3. See a doctor, if needed.
4. Ask someone else who has or has had, a similar issue, to see what they have tried and what has been helpful to them.
5. Do what is required to get better.
6. Get physical activity/rehab without making the issue worse.
7. Adjust what and how much you eat/drink. Try to get 32 oz of water per day.
8. Swap alcohol for special non-alcoholic drinks you will enjoy.
9. Research/consider nutrients like Omega 3's, Vitamin D, Magnesium, Vitamin C, etc.

Ask Yourself: How much of this is due to <u>not being in a relationship with w/someone special</u>?

1. Pray. Ask God for what you want and for direction.
2. Attend a class, an event, or church to meet new people.
3. Ask someone you like to do something with you or help them with something.
4. Ask friends/family if they know someone who might be interested in meeting you.

Ask yourself if it's due to <u>too many people suffering or needing help around you</u>?

1. Pray. Ask God for Wisdom. Pray for whenever/whoever comes to your mind. Ask God to let you know if there is something specific God wants you to do for them and do whatever he says and when. Otherwise, let it go.
2. Limit Facebook time. Let others be responsible for themselves or find someone else to help them. Arrange specific times that work for you to interact with others. Schedule downtime to take care of yourself and do something fun.

3. When someone asks or needs something of you, do what you can without putting yourself at risk or causing problems for yourself.
4. Say "No" when you want/need to (in a loving way!) Only say "Yes," when you want to.

Ask Yourself: How much of this is due to a bad habit?

1. Talk to God. Acknowledge the habit and ask for forgiveness. Ask for wisdom and help in making changes. Pray for your God to keep you from temptation and deliver you from evil each day. Be thankful and count your blessings.
2. Create a Specific Simple Plan
3. Write an Affirmation. Place it on your bathroom mirror, in your phone with a reminder alarm, or your car "dash-board." Say it out loud for 1-2 minutes a day.
4. Come up with a replacement activity or technique to reduce the habit.
5. Set Goals and Reward your progress!
6. Keep away from temptation such as stores, candy aisle, certain websites, keep yourself busy with other activities, eat

with your non-dominate hand, increase your water or vegetable intake, read the bible, etc.
7. Select someone who will help you be accountable and who will encourage you.

Ask Yourself: How much of this is due to spiritual oppression (the devil)?

1. Pray. Then say, "I resist a spirit of depression, gluttony, infirmity, fear, greed, jealousy, or idolatry, etc., and oppression, in the name of Jesus Christ." Say, "Satan, you must go and not return to me in the name of Jesus Christ!" Then ask God to replace what had been taken, with a spirit of joy, peace, health, courage, generosity, faithfulness, and freedom, in the Name of Jesus Christ."
2. Thank God for it.
3. Trust it to be taken care of and do something in faith that lines up with what you have asked God for.

Chapter 6

Dealing with Anger

Dealing with anger is something an individual with bipolar will require, due to high irritability being part of the disease. Also, the judgments and behavior of others may trigger anger for the person. The Following is reference help for dealing with anger.

Dealing with Anger (by Bonnie Bair of Life Improvements, PLLC, 2019)

Anger is a warning indicator light like your engine light on your vehicle. It requires immediate acknowledgment and attention. It's like an alarm. If you ignore it, bad things can happen. For example, if you ignore your alarm clock, you might be late for work and get fired. If you ignore a fire alarm, you may get burned. (In rare instances, it may be important to ignore if the anger response has become a habit or gets worse with attention).

Alarms are created and set for a reason. Anger is our/others' alarm system.

The alarm of anger signifies there is imminent danger of a perceived or real threat to a system –

internal or external. Anger is valid and requires acknowledgment and attention.

Unexplained or frequent uncontrolled anger usually signifies:

A. **When something is going on within the system itself.**

- More than likely it's an internal support system in which internal nutrients are depleted and the body is not functioning as it's designed. It is malfunctioning and is especially sensitive to certain triggering stimuli and the person is more susceptible to stress.

- *Replenish Nutrients Supplies and the internal system will heal.*

B. **When Anger happens with a _Particular Stimuli_** - This signifies an Adjustment in Perception or Communication is needed.

Ask yourself:

1. **Is it due to continual ignorance of either internal or external warning indicator lights?**

-Not listening to God.
-Not listening to self.
-Not listening to others.

2. **Is it due to:** Not asking?   Not telling?
   Not caring?   Not repenting/apologizing?
   Being too busy?   Too much commotion?
   Too many distractions?   Too many
   interruptions?

3. **Is it due to unexpected internal or external warning lights and your perception of it as bad** and because of the perception, you panic or someone else panics.

   How much of this is due to:

   a. Unpreparedness
   b. Being upset because you did not ask God, in the first place.
   c. Not listening to yourself, someone else, or God?
   d. Frustration – due to someone perceiving you as bad or yourself perceiving someone else as bad, or a situation as bad.

e. Misunderstanding – of what God or others say. Or someone misunderstanding what you said or meant.

When Anger Occurs
1. Stop and Assess the Cause/s of Anger
2. Make sure internal systems are working properly
3. Replenish or store up supplies
    - Consider nutrients such as omega 3's, Vitamins, eating different foods, Herbs for dealing with stress such as Holy Basil or Ashwagandha.
    - Do your research!
    - Ask an Expert

4. The body is the temple of the Holy Spirit. Take care of it.
5. Practice Relaxation/Energizing techniques such as Breathing strategies & Kegels
6. Practice Clear Purposeful Thinking

7. Prepare for or avoid specific triggers.

8. Meditate on God's word/Ask God for direction and permission.

9. Follow the plan

10. Adjust, when needed - with your team

- You and God
- You, Spouse & God
- You, God & Family
- You, God, and Team

You cannot serve both God and man, or you will hate the one and love the other. Matthew 6:24

As you serve God, the rest falls into place. Follow God's word and God's direction. Ask God for help and wisdom. Do your best. If something happens unexpectedly, ask God what to do before proceeding. Wait for an answer. (Ask God to help you learn to listen and obey God.)

If something happens unexpectedly and requires emergent action - Call out to God, immediately!

If there is a difference in opinion between you and someone else, stop and ask God. Do not do something you are not okay with or that you are unwilling to do! You have permission to say "No."

There is a reason for the unwillingness. Ask God or the other person to address your concern, before agreeing or proceeding. Be willing to address God's and the other person/s concerns, as well.

When Anger happens in response to <u>frequent stimuli,</u> that happens at <u>expected and unexpected times</u>.

Prepare ahead of time!

1. Your thinking
2. Your response strategy

Examples:

If you prepare for others being clueless or inconsiderate, you will not get as upset as if you expect them not to.

If you prepare for losing track of your keys or phone, you will pay more attention to where you put them, or you will assign them a special place where you can easily find them and make a habit of placing them there regularly.

If you prepare for misunderstandings and for doing something difficult together, you will communicate more clearly and kindly with those around you.

If you prepare for hunger/crabbiness, you will make a shopping list ahead of time and arrange a time to get groceries.

If you have tended to run out of money before payday, you will figure out bills/expenses and establish priorities ahead of spending your paycheck on other things or you might seek a better paying job.

C. **When anger happens in response to frequent ignoring or lack of cooperation. If you've tended to get angry with others because they haven't typically listened or cooperated with you:**

    1. Talk with God about it. Ask God for wisdom and direction.
    2. Proceed with what comes to mind afterward.
    3. If nothing comes to mind.
        a. Talk to the person/people about this.
        b. Ask them what you might do adjust and gain their ear so they can listen/or cooperate with you.

c. Tell them you will be willing to continue to listen and cooperate with them, as they are willing to listen and cooperate with you.
d. Consider doing something different than usual, that gets their attention. Surprise them with a gift or special act of service or outing
e. Try speaking the love language of the other person.
f. If you have spoken their love language and they continue to show little to no interest in speaking yours, they are spoiled. Try telling them you will do x or won't do x if they continue to have disrespected you. Then follow through with your warning.

D. If someone frequently gets snippy with you and this causes you anger:

1. Pray first – Ask God for help and wisdom. Ask God to correct and prepare the person for conversation.
2. Ask the person about their expectations, such as their likes/dislikes/preferences
3. Establish fencing – so you know the rules.
4. Communicate your needs/concerns
5. Look for and negotiate win/win solutions.
   a. Goal of each person
   b. Find a way that's acceptable to both of you. (There are usually multiple ways to get places.) Take turns, if needed.
   c. Ask for help, if necessary.
6. As or after you build the fence, write down the rules for reference so you don't forget. This will establish peace, trust, and enjoyment.

Chapter 7

Emergent Plan for Crisis

Preparing ahead of time will lessen the stress for everyone in the case of a major manic or depressive episode.

A 3-5 step plan specific to the person's needs should be readily accessible to both the individual and family. It should be easy to find in the "Wellness Box."

An example of an emergent plan:

1. Pray with me
2. Lessen expectations of me
3. Ask me to take an Ambien and/or Lithium and get some sleep
4. Schedule an appointment with my doctor
5. *Remember to be honest and kind.*

Chapter 8

To Hospitalize or Not?

It is usually much better to get the person help without going to the hospital. The hospitals have been known to be abusive and insensitive in the treatment of individuals with bipolar disorder by abusing their power for monetary gain. Avoid the hospitals and use them as a last resort only! The trauma a person may endure from a hospital stay may only make things worse for the individual and your relationship - not to mention a person's "pocketbook." The bill for a hospital stay will be astounding! – even with insurance.

A 3-week hospital stay will cost around $68,000. Once a person is admitted into the hospital, they are at the mercy of the hospital and the hospital staff/policies. If you have insurance, plan on staying a minimum of 10 days. Staff decides on your length of stay. If an individual or family member wants them out sooner, it will not matter. The hospital can keep a person for any length of time that they can justify. The person can be held unnecessarily for quite a time. It can feel like a prison. All rights are thrown out the window.

The individual will be treated like an inmate and be housed in rooms next to the opposite sex with individuals that can have violent tendencies or who have illicit drugs in their system.   If a person has insurance, they may end up staying longer than most individuals. This is because staff can count on insurance money. They just need to justify the need to do so in their records - either honestly or dishonestly.

A diagnosis of bipolar disorder often breeds fear of violence, whether there is any history of violence or not. Ignorance and fear of bipolar disorder often result in the person being treated biasedly and unfairly. This can be traumatic and infuriating to the person with bipolar disorder and leads to unfair treatment.

It can snowball for the person with bipolar disorder. And they will be left with little rights and have a mountain of prejudice to overcome, simply because of ignorance (on the part of family and professionals).

The sad thing is that family and professionals are a part of the problem and can exacerbate symptoms for the individual. Family members may be resistant to change habits that have caused stress for the individual. Family may also resent the person with bipolar disorder drawing attention to the need for change within the family system and the person with the bi-polar disorder may often become the scapegoat for the family. It's easier to label the individual as crazy than to take responsibility and change unhealthy habits that affect the relationship and subsequently the individual.

Professionals contribute to the problem by not knowing enough about alternative support therapies including alternatives to medication - such as CBD, flaxseed oil and ashwagandha, etc.

Professionals and families can be quick to get law enforcement involved, rather than use good judgment and compromise. This sets up distrust and resentment and further trauma for the individual.

Healthy limits and respect of all individuals involved are necessary for fair and effective treatment. To treat the individual with bipolar disorder and not the sick system leaves an unnecessary burden on the individual. It also leads to future problems for them and their families. Education and treatment options are essential!

It is common for family members to lie to an individual to coerce them into treatment facilities where more abuse takes place. Families need to learn to cooperate. Rather than individuals or family members expecting cooperation to be one-sided, families must adopt methods of two-sided cooperation. This would keep abusive situations from happening and would be motivating for individuals to get help sooner, rather than later. When family members abuse their power and lie to a member for coercion or lie to a hospital or law enforcement official for getting the family member some help, this only creates resentment and destroys the spirit of the individual and it strains the relationship of the family. It should not be so difficult to get help! Medical and Law Enforcement professionals need to be better educated for assisting in the humane treatment of individuals with bipolar disorder!

Even psychiatrists are ill-equipped at times. Needed medicines often have problematic side effects. Psychiatrists often prescribe medicines without checking on nutritional deficiencies. Often doctors prescribe antidepressants when they should be prescribing mood stabilizers with anti-depressant properties. These things can ruin the lives of the people they are supposed to be serving. They may even threaten to call the police on the person that is unwilling to take a particular type of medication. There needs to be better coping and assisting strategies for helping individuals with bipolar disorder. Do your best to address both their concerns, as well as your own, and you will be more successful.

Often individuals with bipolar disorder may just need a break from the situation or environment they are living in. There need to be other options for people besides going to a hospital in which their situation ultimately becomes worse. If people are stressed because of finances etc. and they can't afford counseling, going to the hospital is surely not going to fix things. It may make their family feel better temporarily, but it typically does not make things better, nor is it the best way of handling things.

Families are deceived if they think it is wise to lie about their family members for them to get help. I have known cases in which professionals were told a person was being violent so they could get them locked away in the hospital for "treatment." The main problem with this is that the person is liable to be put on the wrong medication, because of this untrue report. Thus, continuing future problems and more unfair/inaccurate treatment and abuse of power.

I believe the reason the system doesn't change is that:

> **1)** it is easier for families to scapegoat and medicate than it is for them to apologize and change behavior.

> **2)** It is more profitable for medical professionals to medicate than for them to heal patients.

3) It is thought to be easier for society to lock individuals away and medicate, rather than take time to listen and attend to a problem when it arises.

4) it is more profitable for farmers to use farming practices that contaminate and strip the land of important nutrients needed for mental health.

Medication is helpful and often necessary to help people to deal with the stresses at hand. However, it is all too often the first and only go to. And maybe the wrong medication for the person.

I have found that individuals who are resistant to taking medications, due to issues with being sensitive or allergic to medications, are much more vulnerable. This falls in line with their heightened sensitivity to people and situations (common in people with bipolar disorder). They need something to help support their body and emotions. Some nutrients can support them.

However, if these were made known to patients, patients would not have to keep going to the doctor for medication refills and it would ultimately hurt the income of doctors.

Chapter 9

Advice for Family/Individual

Advice for Family

A family should do its best to be kind and truthful and to avoid lying and trickery. It will hurt your relationship and tick off your family member. It will incite more anger and make matters worse and recovery longer.

Communicate with your loved one and know what to do in the case of an emergent situation.

Follow the Plan!

Do your best to be healthy yourself.

Advice for the Individual

Do your best to stay on top of your health yourself. When things start to tilt or spin out of control, follow your plan, and speak with professionals, as needed. The priority is getting adequate sleep and regular meals/exercise. You know your needs, listen to the voice inside, don't brush things off or be too proud to ask for help or to take medicine.

Make a "Wellness Box" for your reference, to include anything you may need to help avoid or manage a manic/depressive episode.

Make a 3 to 5 step emergency plan that is easy for you and everyone else to follow. Make sure to have it easily accessible to family /or close friends. Doing so will help to ensure things are taken care of in the way you prefer.

Follow the Plan!

3-5 Step Emergent Plan

*How everyone responds in a difficult situation is dependent on everyone's mental health, as well as the individual with bipolar disorder. It is also dependent on their ability to change their habits and biases. A clear simple plan is best, to ensure it is followed.

Sample Emergent Plan

1. Pray
2. Lessen responsibilities
3. Sleeping pill and or lithium
4. Call Doctor.

Chapter 10

Summary

Having bipolar disorder is not a sin or something to be ashamed of. Bipolar disorder is usually always inherited. Research shows head injury can also contribute to bipolar disorder. It is often misunderstood, undiagnosed, and inadequately treated. However, it requires accurate and adequate treatment for successful functioning in life and for enjoying satisfying relationships.

The craziness in this world adds stress to persons with bipolar disorder; making the disease more difficult to manage since individuals with bipolar disorder can be extremely sensitive to external, as well as internal stimuli.

The stigma of having bipolar disorder is often unfair and difficult to overcome.

It depends on personality, upbringing, experiences, and situation, etc., as to how a person with bipolar is going to behave. Sometimes a person with bipolar may be the scapegoat or the tyrant in a family. The family can either be insensitive to the individual or walk on "eggshells," around the person – sometimes both.

Healthy communication/cooperation helps manage bipolar disorder; along with adequate medicine/nutrients, eating and sleeping schedules.

Keeping a "Wellness Box" to contain, medicines/nutrients, phone numbers of doctors and friends, affirmations, reference notes for self and others, communication helps, and a 3-5 step emergency plan, are essential for successful bipolar disorder management.

Although there are similarities in characteristics of bipolar disorder, each person is an individual and needs to be treated as such and with respect.

Dealing with bipolar disorder is challenging for all persons involved. Family and close friends have historically been ill-equipped for the challenge it poses. Communication and planning are essential for eliminating fears and adequate respectful treatment. Hopefully, as this happens and through education, the stigma of bipolar disorder will cease, and life will become more pleasant and sane for everyone involved.